The Essentia̲ ̲ ̲ ̲ ̲ ̲ ̲ Protein Cookbook

Protein-Packed and Delicious Recipes
for Dinner

Table of Contents

Introduction **4**

1. Ancho Chicken tacos **5**

2.Spinach and Tomato pasta with poached egg..................**8**

3.Avocado cucumber grapefruit salad **11**

4.Salmon piccata.. **13**

5.Tofu Spinach Sauté **16**

6.Spicy Black Bean Soup................................... **18**

7.Sweet chili rubbed salmon **21**

8.Orecchiette pasta with chicken sausage and broccoli **24**

9.Shrimp tacos **27**

10.Chicken Fajitas **30**

11.Spiced chickpea and broccoli wrap **33**

12.Honey garlic shrimp and broccoli **36**

13.Grilled salmon with avocado bruschetta **38**

14.Taco soup... **41**

15.Tilapia with tomato and broccoli.................... **43**

16.Grilled cheese with Brussels sprouts and pear............ **45**

17.Chicken and veggie stir-fry **47**

18.Maple and mustard grilled chicken..................... **49**

19.Pea and Farro Stir-Fry................................ **51**

20.Chickpea Tikka Masala **53**

21.Kale and Sweet Potato Quesadilla..................... **56**

22.Chicken lettuce wraps with miso-peanut oil 58

23.Shrimp Caesar spinach salad 61

24.Vegan Lo Mein 65

25.Kale salad with Caesar dressing and avocado 68

26.Sheet pan salmon 71

27.Jalapeno popper chicken 74

28.Sheet pan dinner 76

29.Black Bean and Corn salad 79

30.Ground beef veggie skillet 81

Conclusion 84

Introduction

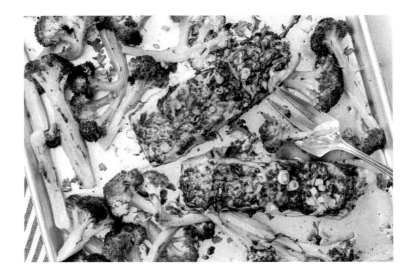

If you have ever heard of the Atkins diet, then you know that one of the fundamentals of the diet is to eat lots of protein in place of carbohydrates. The protein-rich food is especially helpful if you are working out while dieting because it allows the body to break down fat and build muscle faster. The protein in your diet will also help you feel fuller for longer so you experience a decrease in appetite without noticing any hunger pangs. Some of the recipes in this book are high-protein dishes with a small amount of carbohydrates thrown in for filler. You can enjoy these recipes with or without the bread included, it is completely up to you.

1. Ancho Chicken tacos

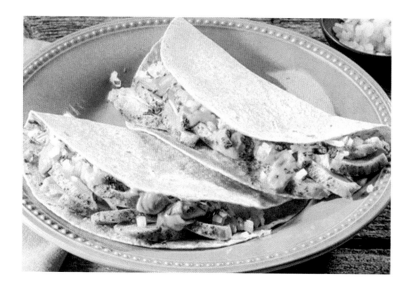

These tacos are one of my favourite recipes to serve to my family. Try these with some delicious garnishes like lime, sour cream, avocado, red onions or jalapenos.

Preparation Time-10 minutes

Servings-12

Ingredients

tacos

- 12 small corn tortillas
- 2-3 shredded green cabbage leaves

- 1 chopped bunch cilantro
- ancho chicken
- 4 ounces all-purpose flour
- 1/3 ounce ancho chili powder
- 1 teaspoon taco seasoning
- 1 pinch of salt and pepper
- 1 ounce oil
- 24 ounces boneless skinless chicken breasts, quartered

Directions

1. Place cabbage cilantro in a mixing bowl and toss well.

2. In a shallow dish, flour, chili powder, seasoning, salt and pepper

3. Heat oil in a pan on Medium High heat

4. In a heavy duty pan, heat the oil on medium high heat. Dredge chicken pieces in flour mixture and place in hot oil.

5. Cook chicken quarters for 1-2 minutes per side until cooked through and browned

6. Remove chicken from heat and set aside until cool enough to handle. Season with salt and shred with two forks.

7. Place tortillas in the microwave for 10-20 seconds and serve with chicken and your favourite toppings.

2.Spinach and Tomato pasta with poached egg

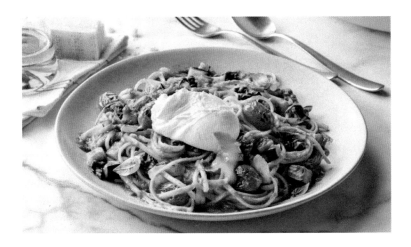

Preparation Time-10 minutes

Servings-12

Ingredients

- 2 ounces whole wheat penne, uncooked
- ½ ounce olive oil
- 2 cored medium beefsteak tomatoes, chopped
- Salt and pepper
- 8 ounces baby spinach, loosely packed
- ½ ounce grated Parmesan cheese
- 1 ounce nutritional yeast flakes

- ¼ teaspoon paprika
- 1 ounce chopped fresh basil, chopped
- 1 egg

Directions

Bring a pot of water to a boil and then cook the pasta according to package instructions. Drain and set aside.

Heat oil in a large frying pan on Medium Low. Sauté tomatoes in the oil and season with salt and pepper.

Cook for 10 minutes, stirring frequently until tomatoes are broken down and softened

Add yeast and spinach to the tomatoes and season with paprika

Cook and stir until spinach wilts. Pour cooked penne into the pan and season with basil. Reduce heat to Low.

In a small bowl, crack egg keeping the yolk intact

Heat 5" of water in a small pan on Medium Low and bring it to a simmer. Stir water until a gently whirlpool forms in the pan and drop egg into the middle of the whirlpool.

Poach for 3-4 minutes and remove from water with a slotted spoon.

Place egg on top of the penne and sprinkle with parmesan cheese

3.Avocado cucumber grapefruit salad

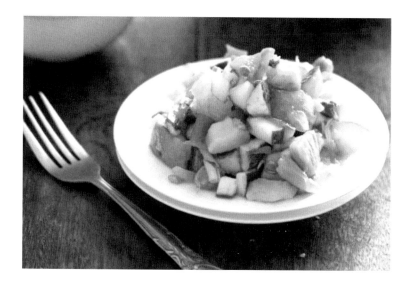

I like to serve this salad with some shaved almonds sprinkled generously on top. The refreshing flavour of the fresh vegetables and fruit make this salad a great summer snack.

Preparation Time-20 minutes

Servings-4

Ingredients

salad

- 16 ounces diced cucumbers, with seeds removed
- 16 ounces peeled orange, chopped

- 12 ounces diced avocado
- 2 ½ ounces chopped smoked almonds
- 1 ounce chopped fresh mint
- 2 ounces chopped fresh chives

dressing

- ½ ounce fresh lemon juice
- ¾ ounce honey
- ¾ ounce olive oil
- orange zest
- salt

Directions

1. Toss all of the **salad Ingredients** in a large mixing bowl until fully combined.

2. Whisk lemon juice, honey, olive oil, orange zest and salt in a small bowl and drizzle over the **salad** to taste.

3. Place in the refrigerator to chill before serving.

4.Salmon piccata

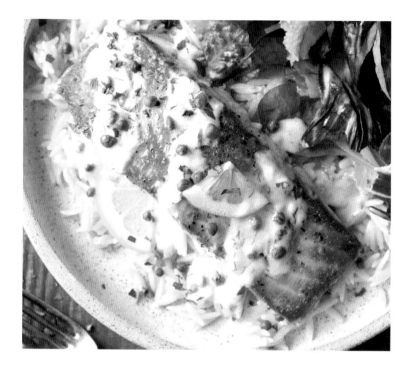

I prepare meals for the week on Sundays and then store them in the refrigerator or freeze them. This piccata always makes it into the week's rotation.

Preparation Time-20 minutes

Servings-4

Ingredients

- 4 x 8-ounce salmon fillets
- Kosher salt
- black pepper, freshly ground
- 5 ounces all-purpose flour, divided
- 1 ounce olive oil
- 1 ounce butter
- 2 minced cloves garlic
- 2 ounces white wine
- 8 ounces chicken stock
- 1 juiced lemon
- 1/2 thinly sliced lemon
- 2 ounces capers
- 1 ounce sun-dried tomatoes, finely chopped
- 1 ounce parsley, freshly chopped

Directions

1. Pour flour into a shallow dish. Sprinkle salmon with salt and pepper and dredge in the flour. Shake salmon gently to remove any excess flour.

2. Heat olive oil in a large frying pan on medium heat. Sear salmon for 4-5 minutes per side until golden. Place salmon on a plate and tent with aluminum foil to keep the fish warm.

3. Melt butter in a wide pan and sauté garlic in the butter for 1-2 minutes until fragrant. Whisk flour into the mixture for 1-2 minutes until a light gold colour.

4. Gently whisk in white wine and scrape any food particles left at the bottom of the frying pan as you cook.

5. Add stock and whisk until combined. Cook for 4-5 minutes at a simmer.

6. Stir in the rest of the **Ingredients** except for parsley and place salmon in the sauce in the pan. Cook for 3-4 minutes. Top with parsley before serving.

5.Tofu Spinach Sauté

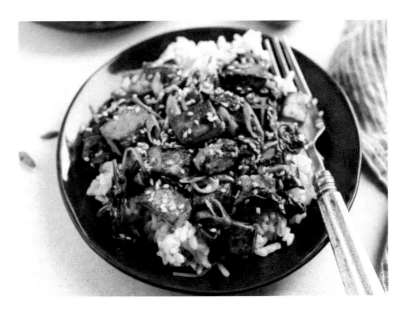

Try this delicious spinach sauté when you are looking for a meatless protein-packed meal. I love using extra sriracha for a spicy treat.

Preparation Time-10 minutes

Servings-2

Ingredients

- 2 ounces onion, chopped
- 2 ounces button mushrooms, chopped
- 8 ounces pressed extra-firm tofu, diced in 1" pieces

- ½ ounce nutritional yeast
- 1 teaspoon coconut aminos
- 32 ounces baby spinach
- 5 chopped grape tomatoes
- cooking spray
- sriracha sauce

Directions

1. Coat a non-stick frying pan with cooking spray on medium heat. Sauté mushrooms and onions for 2-3 minutes until tender.

2. Toss tofu in with the onions and mushrooms and onions for 2-3 minutes.

3. Stir in coconut aminos and yeast until well combined and mixture is coated fully

4. Add spinach and tomatoes to the pan and cook for 3-4 minutes until spinach starts to wilt.

5. Serve topped with sriracha

6.Spicy Black Bean Soup

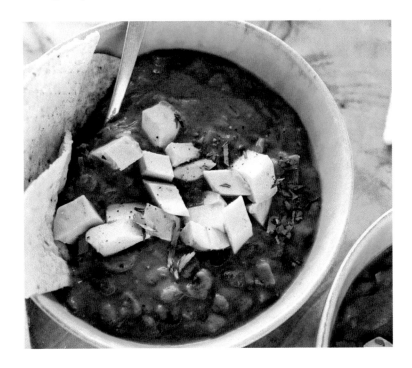

This delicious soup also tastes amazing with some shredded Tex-Mex cheese liberally sprinkled on top. If you want it creamier, add sour cream.

Preparation Time-7 minutes

Servings-2

Ingredients

- ½ ounce olive oil
- ½ onion, finely diced
- 2 clove garlic, minced
- 1 red bell pepper, diced
- 15 ½ ounce can black beans, rinsed and drained
- 8 ½ ounces vegetable broth
- 1 ½ ounces fresh cilantro, chopped
- 1 ½ teaspoon ground cumin
- ¼ teaspoon red pepper flakes
- ½ ounce balsamic vinegar
- ½ peeled and pitted avocado, sliced
- 2 tortillas
- 1 slice cheddar cheese

Directions

Heat olive oil in a large pot on medium heat.

Get a pot and add one tbsp of olive oil.

Sauté onion and garlic in the oil until softened and fragrant

Add bell pepper to the onion and garlic and sauté for 2-3 minutes

Squash a portion of the black beans with a fork and add all of them to the pot

Stir in vegetable broth, cilantro, cumin pepper flakes and vinegar. Simmer for another 10 minutes.

Heat up tortillas and serve soup with sliced avocado, tortillas and a slice of cheddar cheese.

7.Sweet chili rubbed salmon

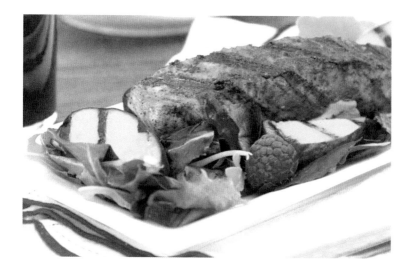

I love serving this delicious rubbed salmon on a bed of quinoa or brown rice. It also tastes just as good with nothing but a fresh, green **salad** and a dash of lemon juice.

Preparation Time-5 minutes

Servings-4

Ingredients

- 4 x 5-ounce wild salmon fillets
- 32 ounces broccolini stems
- 16 ounces cooked quinoa
- ½ ounce fresh dill

- ½ ounce chili powder
- 1 tsp ground cumin
- 1 tsp garlic powder
- ½ tsp onion powder
- 1 tsp powdered stevia extract
- salt and pepper
- 1 lemon, cut into 4 wedges

Directions

1. Preheat the oven to 400 degrees Fahrenheit.

2. Combine dill, chili powder, cumin, garlic, onion powder and stevia extract in a bowl.

3. Arrange salmon on a baking pan covered with foil and season fish with the dill mixture. Evenly distribute dry rub by rubbing the fish with the back of a spoon or your hand.

4. Season salmon with salt and pepper. Cover the fish in foil and bake for 15 minutes until it is easily flaked with a fork

5. In the meantime, place steam insert in a pot of water and steam broccolini until tender. Season with salt and pepper

6. Serve salmon and broccolini on a plate with a splash of lemon juice

8.Orecchiette pasta with chicken sausage and broccoli

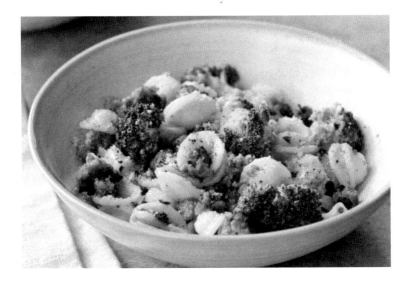

This Orecchiette pasta recipe will hit the spot and give you some much needed protein. You can serve this with some shredded cheese on the side for extra flavor.

Preparation Time-5 minutes

Servings-8

Ingredients

- 14 ounces Italian chicken sausage with casing removed
- 12 ounces uncooked pasta
- 16 ounces fresh broccoli florets, stems removed
- 5 smashed cloves garlic, chopped
- 2 ounces Parmesan cheese, grated
- 1 ounce olive oil, divided
- kosher salt
- fresh cracked pepper

Directions

In a big pot with salted boiling water, cook the pasta according to package instructions and add broccoli when water starts to boil. Cook broccoli and pasta until al dente. Reserve 8 ounces of cooking water and drain.

Heat a large frying pan on medium high heat and brown sausage for 5-7 minutes until it is evenly cooked and crumbly. Break meat up into pieces and remove from heat

Heat ½ ounce of olive oil in the same large pot on High heat. Sauté garlic in the oil for 1 minute until fragrant.

Reduce heat to low and return the pasta to the pot. Add sausage and mix well. Add the remaining **Ingredients** and gently mash large pieces of broccoli.

Add 4 ounces of reserved cooking water or more if needed.

9.Shrimp **tacos**

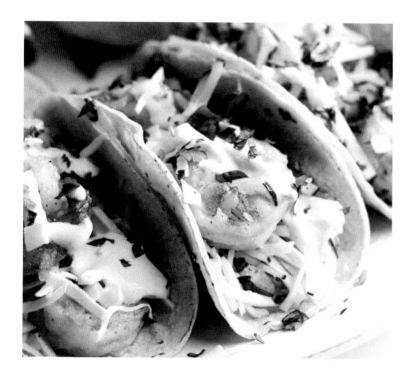

The shrimp **tacos** are delicious and nutritious, not to mention addictive! I have added goat cheese to this mix with amazing results.

Preparation Time-5 minutes

Servings-8

Ingredients

- 4 ounces peeled and cleaned fresh shrimp, tails removed
- Pepper
- Salt
- ¼ teaspoon paprika, divided
- 1/3 ounce canola oil
- 3 small corn tortillas
- 2 ounces fresh corn kernels
- ½ peeled medium ripe mango, chopped
- 1 ounce crumbled feta
- ½ ounce chopped fresh mint leaves
- Zest and juice from ½ lime

Directions

Sprinkle shrimp with 1/8 teaspoon of paprika, pepper and salt until completely covered

Heat oil in a large frying pan on medium heat and sauté shrimp in the oil for 2 minutes per side until opaque.

Remove shrimp from heat and when cool enough to handle, chop roughly.

Wipe the frying pan and return to medium heat. Cook tortillas in the pan for 1 minute per side until warm.

Combine the rest of the **Ingredients** and serve on top of the tortillas.

10.Chicken Fajitas

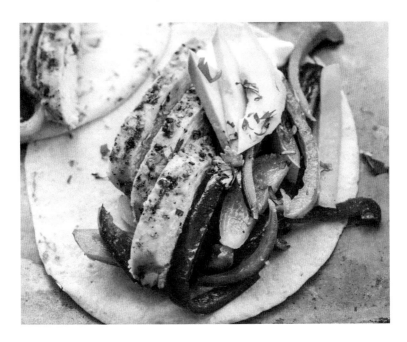

These fajitas are simple to make and fun for the family to eat. I like to experiment with different fillings and add some sriracha sauce when the mood strikes.

Preparation Time-5 minutes

Servings-4

Ingredients

- 16 ounces boneless and skinless chicken breast, sliced into thin strips

- 1 tsp dried oregano
- 1 ounce cilantro, chopped
- 1 tsp chili powder
- ½ tsp ground cumin
- 1 tsp sweet paprika
- 1 minced garlic clove
- 1 tsp fine grain salt, divided
- 1 ounces olive oil, divided
- ½ lime, juiced
- 2 thinly sliced bell peppers
- 1 sliced thin onion

Directions

Toss chicken in a large mixing bowl with oregano, cilantro, chili powder, cumin, paprika, garlic and salt until coated.

Heat ½ ounce of olive oil in a large frying pan on medium high heat. Place peppers in the oil in one layer and char them slightly before stirring gently.

Add onion and half the salt to the pan and wait until onion's are translucent before mixing them. Transfer mixture to a plate and scrape frying pan to clear.

Heat the rest of the olive oil in the same frying pan on medium heat. Add chicken to the oil in a single layer and brown on one side. Flip chicken over and continue to cook and flip for 6 minutes until both browned evenly

Return pepper mixture to the pan and add lime juice. Heat mixture and sprinkle with cilantro before serving

11.Spiced chickpea and broccoli wrap

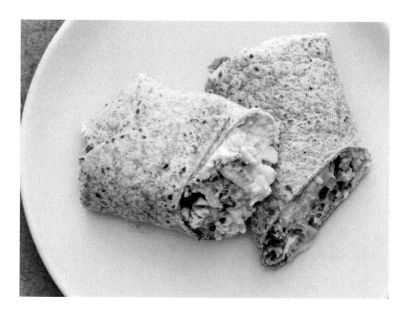

This wrap makes a delicious meat-free snack that is protein-packed and filling. You can substitute butter lettuce leaves for the tortilla if you want to decrease your carb intake.

Preparation Time-15 minutes

Servings-1

Ingredients

- 1 tsp olive oil, divided
- 8 ounces broccoli florets
- Salt
- Pepper
- 6 ounces rinsed and drained canned chickpeas
- 1 ounce nutritional yeast flakes
- 1 crumbled ounce goat cheese
- ½ ounce vegetable stock
- ¼ tsp cumin
- ½ ounce chopped fresh parsley
- 10" whole-wheat tortilla

Directions

Heat oil in a small frying pan on medium heat. Cook broccoli in the oil for 5-6 minutes until al dente. Season with salt and pepper.

Combine yeast, chickpeas, stock, goat cheese and cumin in a microwaveable bowl. Sprinkle with salt and pepper and cook on high for 1 minute. Stir mixture and cook for another 1 minute.

Remove from microwave and parsley. Mash mixture with a fork gently.

Warm the tortilla in the microwave and scoop chickpea mixture onto the middle of the tortilla. Top with broccoli, wrap and serve

12.Honey garlic shrimp and broccoli

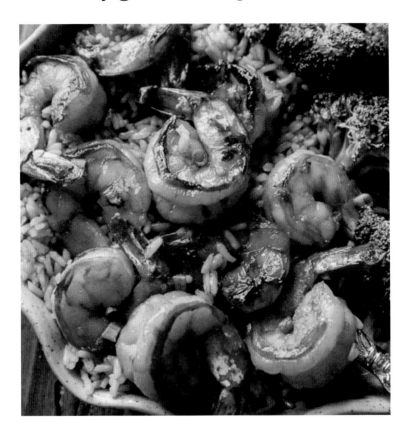

This delicious combination of sweet and savoury tastes even better over a bed of cauliflower rice or quinoa. Use fresh jumbo shrimp if you can for a big juicy taste!

Preparation Time-15 minutes

Servings-4

Ingredients

- 16 ounces peeled and deveined jumbo shrimp
- 8 ounces frozen broccoli florets
- ½ ounce oil
- For the Sauce
- 1 teaspoon minced garlic
- ½ teaspoon minced ginger
- 2 ounces honey
- 1 ½ ounces soy sauce

Directions

Place broccoli in a mixing bowl with 1/3 ounce of water and cook in a microwaveable bowl for 2 minutes on high.

Whisk sauce **Ingredients** together and split in half

Place shrimp in half of the sauce and marinate overnight.

Heat oil in a frying pan on high heat. Sear marinated shrimp for 1-2 minutes per side until browned

Add broccoli and drizzle with the rest of the sauce.

13.Grilled salmon with avocado bruschetta

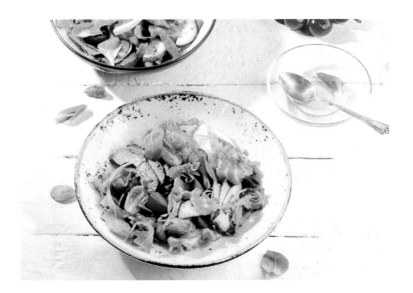

When you think bruschetta, you automatically think bread. Not so with this amazing and simple bread-less meal.

Preparation Time-15 minutes

Servings-4

Ingredients

- cooking spray
- 4 (6-ounce) wild salmon filets
- 1/4 teaspoon kosher salt

- black pepper
- Avocado bruschetta
- 2 ounces red onion, chopped
- ½ ounce extra virgin oil
- ½ ounce balsamic vinegar
- kosher salt
- fresh cracked pepper
- 2 vine ripe tomatoes, chopped
- 2 minced cloves garlic
- 1 ounce chopped fresh basil leaves
- 4 ounces avocado, diced

Directions

Mix oil, vinegar, kosher salt and pepper in a large mixing bowl and let stand for 5 minutes.

Add tomatoes to the bowl and mix.

Mix in garlic, basil, and more salt and pepper to taste. Set mixture aside for 10-15 minutes

Preheat grill and lightly coat grates with cooking spray.

Sprinkle salmon with salt and pepper until fully coated and place on the grill with the skin facing down

Close the grill lid and cook for 8-10 minutes without opening.

Remove salmon and cover with tin foil. Let stand for 2-3 minutes.

Add diced avocado to the bruschetta and serve salmon with equal amounts of bruschetta mixture.

14.Taco soup

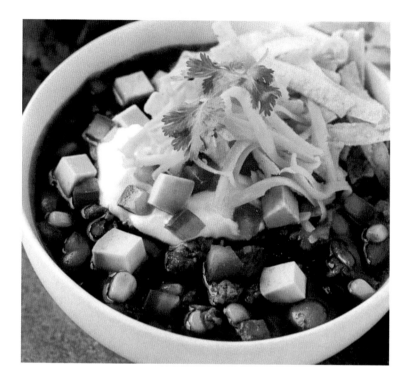

I heap on the shredded cheese when I have this soup because it tastes so creamy and delicious. This also tastes great with some sour cream mixed in.

Preparation Time-15 minutes

Servings-4

Ingredients

- 16 ounces extra-lean ground beef
- 1 chopped onion
- 38 ounces rinsed canned black beans
- 19 ounces canned diced tomatoes, undrained
- 14 ounces tomato sauce
- 8 ounces frozen corn
- 1 ¼ ounce taco seasoning mix
- 16 ounces water
- 8 ounces Shredded Tex Mex Cheese

Directions

In a large pan, combine meat and onions. Cook until meat is evenly browned and onions are translucent. Drain.

Add black beans, tomatoes, tomato sauce, corn, seasoning mix and water to the pan and bring mixture to a boil.

Reduce heat to medium low and simmer for 5 minutes.

15.Tilapia with tomato and broccoli

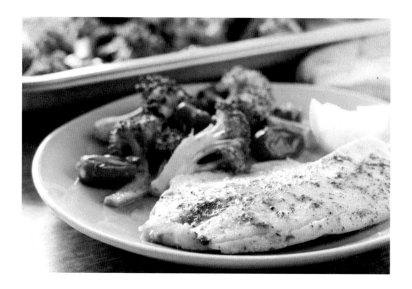

The refreshing tangy taste of the tomatoes complement the mild taste of the tilapia. I like to serve this on quinoa as well as rice or even cauliflower rice.

Preparation Time-20 minutes

Servings-2

Ingredients

- 2 x 4oz tilapia fillets
- Salt
- Pepper

- 20 cherry tomatoes, cut in half
- 16 ounces broccoli florets
- 6 thinly sliced cloves garlic
- 2 ounces torn fresh parsley
- 1 ounce olive oil
- 1/3 ounce soy sauce
- 1/3 ounce unseasoned rice vinegar
- 12 ounces warmed cooked brown rice

Directions

Heat oven to 400 degrees Fahrenheit

Line a baking sheet with parchment paper.

Sprinkle fillets with salt and pepper on both sides. Arrange tilapia, broccoli, tomatoes, parsley and garlic on one side of the parchment paper.

Pour soy sauce, oil and vinegar over the mixture and fold the parchment into a packet, seal edges

Bake for 10-12 minutes. Remove from heat and let cool for 2 minutes. Serve tilapia mixture on a bed of brown rice

16.Grilled cheese with Brussels sprouts and pear

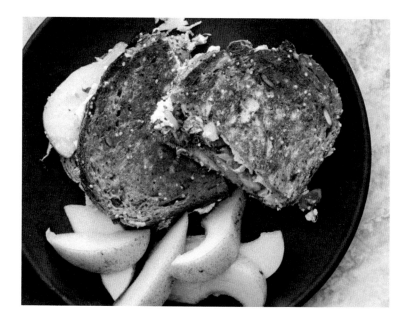

The pear adds a lovely fresh taste to this grilled cheese sandwich you can't resist. I like to add some Tex Mex cheese when I want a spicier kick.

Preparation Time-20 minutes

Servings-2

Ingredients

- 1 tsp olive oil, divided
- 3 thinly sliced brussels sprouts
- 2 slices whole-wheat bread
- 1 ounce room-temperature goat cheese
- ½ cored and thinly sliced medium pear, divided
- 1 ounce grated Parmesan cheese

Directions

Heat ½ teaspoon of olive oil in a frying pan. Sauté Brussels sprouts in the oil for 2 minutes until bright green and tender. Remove from pan and set aside

Spread a slice of whole-wheat bread with softened goat cheese. Arrange layers on the bread by adding Brussels sprouts, followed by half of the pear, then parmesan cheese.

Wipe the frying pan and heat the rest of the olive oil. Cook sandwich in the oil for 3 minutes per side, until toasted and cheese melts.

Serve with rest of pear

17.Chicken and veggie stir-fry

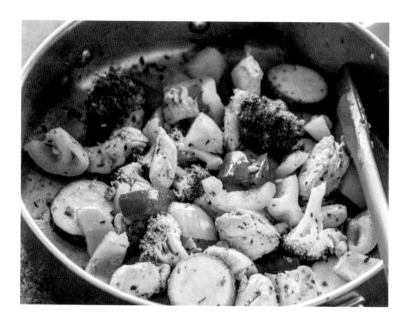

This stir-fry tastes amazing with a fresh green **salad** or served on a bed of brown rice or quinoa. If you prefer a heartier meal, then try it with a small portion of pasta or garlic bread.

Preparation Time-10 minutes

Servings-4

Ingredients

- 1 ounce olive oil
- 16 ounces boneless skinless chicken breasts, slice into ½" piece
- 16 ounces broccoli florets
- 1 large sliced zucchini
- 1 medium sliced bell peppers, cut in ½" pieces
- 1 medium sliced yellow onion cut in half and ½" pieces
- 4 cloves crushed garlic
- ½ ounce Italian seasoning
- 1 teaspoon salt
- ½ teaspoon black pepper

Directions

1. Heat 1 ounce of oil in a large frying pan on medium-high heat.

2. Sauté all of the **Ingredients** in the oil for 8-10 minutes until vegetables are tender and chicken is no longer pink inside.

18.Maple and mustard grilled chicken

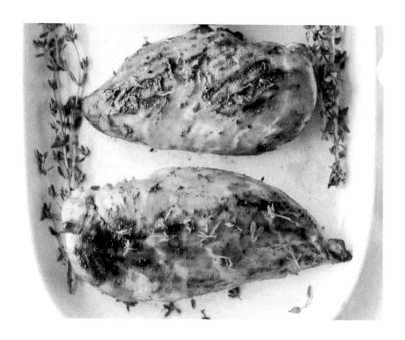

This unique chicken recipe tastes even better when served with some sweet-potato fries. These make the perfect BBQ snack in the summer when you have people over.

Preparation Time-10 minutes

Servings-4

Ingredients

- 16 ounces chicken breast tenders, cut in 1" chunks
- 4 ounces honey mustard dressing
- 1 sliced red onion, chopped into 1" pieces
- Bamboo skewers soaked in water for 2 hours

Directions

1. Preheat grill on High.

2. Combine chicken and onion in a mixing bowl. Add dressing and toss until chicken and onions are coated.

3. Cook skewer on grill for 9-12 minutes until heated through. Rotate halfway through to evenly cook.

4. Remove skewers from grill and serve.

19.Pea and Farro Stir-Fry

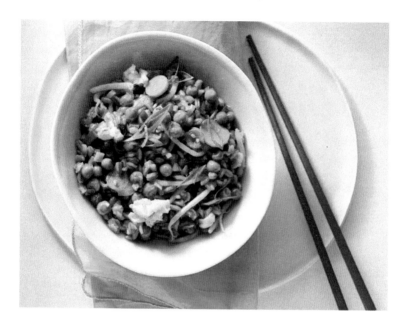

Serve this delicious stir-fry over a bed of cauliflower rice or quinoa for a protein-packed meal. If you want to add a little spice, try sriracha sauce.

Preparation Time-10 minutes

Servings-4

Ingredients

- 1/3 ounce olive oil, divided
- 2 large beaten eggs

- ½ thinly sliced medium sweet onion
- Salt
- Pepper
- 2 minced cloves garlic
- 5 ½ ounces cooked farro
- 8 ounces fresh peas
- ¼ teaspoon paprika
- 2 ounces torn fresh basil

Directions

Heat 1 teaspoon of olive oil in a large cast-iron frying pan on medium high heat

Stir eggs into oil and don't stop stirring for 30 seconds until eggs are cooked. Remove eggs to a plate.

Place frying pan on medium heat and heat up the rest of the olive oil. Sauté onion in the oil for 5 minutes until tender.

Add garlic and sauté for 1 minute until fragrant. Seasons with salt and pepper

Stir in the rest of the **Ingredients** including the cooked egg and mix until well combined and heated through

20.Chickpea Tikka Masala

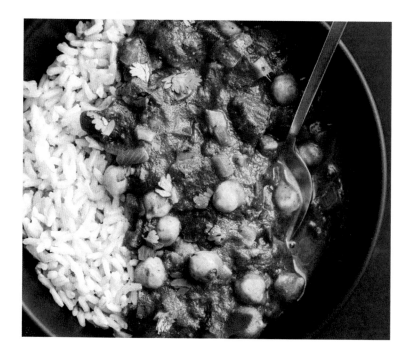

Chickpeas are full of protein so this recipe will give you something tasty to nibble on and will fulfill your protein intake. The herbs and spices in this dish are heavenly and addictive!

Preparation Time-10 minutes

Servings-8

Ingredients

- 1 ounces olive oil
- 1 large finely chopped onion
- 2 minced garlic cloves
- 2" finely chopped piece of ginger
- ½ ounce Garam Masala
- 1/3 ounce ground coriander
- 1/3 ounce ground cumin
- 1/3 ounce paprika
- 1 teaspoon turmeric
- ½ teaspoon cayenne pepper
- 3 x 15 ounces canned chickpeas, drained and rinsed
- 2 x 14 ½ ounces cans diced tomatoes
- 13 ½ ounces can full fat coconut milk
- 1 teaspoon cornstarch
- Salt
- Chopped cilantro

Directions

Heat oil in a large pan on medium high heat. Add a pinch of salt to the oil and sauté onions in the pan for 6 minutes until translucent. Stir occasionally.

Sauté garlic in the oil for 1 minute until fragrant. Add ginger, Garam Masala, coriander, cumin, paprika, turmeric and cayenne and sauté for 30 seconds until fragrant.

Add chickpeas and tomatoes and bring mixture to a boil. Reduce heat and simmer for 15 minutes.

Add coconut milk and cook for another 5 minutes.

Whisk cornstarch and 1 ounce of water in a small bowl until combined. Add cornstarch mixture to the pan and simmer for another 5 minutes until gravy has reached desired consistency.

Remove from heat and serve topped with a sprinkle of cilantro

21.Kale and Sweet Potato Quesadilla

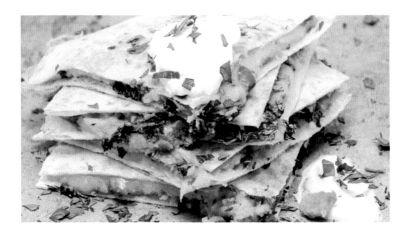

The whole wheat tortilla in this recipe makes this protein-infused recipe filling and delicious. I have also tried this as a bread-less meal with some sour cream and sriracha sauce.

Preparation Time-15 minutes

Servings-1

Ingredients

- 1 washed medium sweet potato
- 8 ounces thinly sliced kale leaves
- 1 teaspoon olive oil
- 10" whole-wheat tortilla
- 1 ½ ounces shredded Parmesan cheese

- ½ ounce torn fresh basil

Directions

Poke small holes in the sweet potato with a fork. Wrap it in a dampened paper towel. Place wrapped potato in the microwave for 6 minutes on High heat until tender.

Remove the potato. Once cool enough to handle, remove skin. Mash with a fork or potato masher.

Pour 1" of water into a large frying pan and bring to a simmer on Medium.

Add kale to the water and cook for 3 minutes until soft and wilted. Stir often. Drain and shake kale dry.

Clean out frying pan and place it back on the element on medium low heat. Place 1 tortilla in the pan to heat up. Arrange mashed potato, kale, cheese and basil on half of the tortilla and fold the other half over the filling. Cook for 3 minutes until cheese is melted and flip the tortilla over. Remove from heat when both sides are browned evenly and cheese is completely melted.

Cut into 4 pieces and serve

22.Chicken lettuce wraps with miso-peanut oil

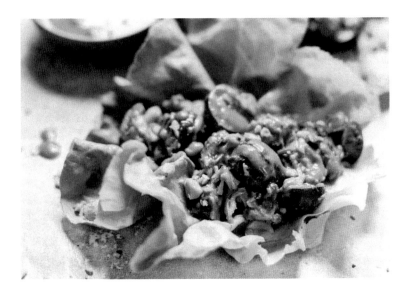

There are so many foods that can substitute for a bread wrap and lettuce is one of the healthiest. I like to serve this with some extra soy on the side.

Preparation Time-15 minutes

Servings-4

Ingredients

Sauce:

- 2 ounces crunchy peanut butter
- 1 ½ ounces miso
- 4 ounces vegetable broth
- ½ ounce soy sauce
- 1 minced clove garlic
- 3 minced green onions
- 1 ribbed and seeded jalapeno, minced
- lettuce wraps
- 16 ounces boneless skinless chicken breasts
- ½ ounce chili powder
- salt and pepper
- 24 ounces grapes, cut in half
- butter lettuce leaves
- lime juice

Directions

1. Whisk peanut butter, miso, broth, soy sauce, garlic, onions and jalapeno together until creamy and smooth

2. Pre-heat a frying pan over medium high heat. Add some butter.

3. Coat chicken with chili powder, salt and pepper and add to the butter in the pan. Cook chicken for 3-4 minutes per side until it is no longer pink inside. Remove chicken from heat and shred with two forks after it has cooled for a minute.

4. Mix half of the peanut butter sauce with chicken and grapes in a large mixing bowl. Add more sauce as required to coat all **Ingredients** fully.

5. Arrange lettuce leaves on a serving plate and stuff each one with chicken mixture. Drizzle some extra sauce on the wrap and serve.

23.Shrimp Caesar spinach **salad**

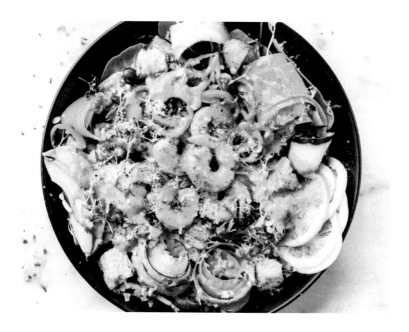

This Caesar **salad** tastes fantastic with some shaved roasted almonds and red pepper flakes. I like to have some fresh shredded parmesan cheese on the table for those who want to splurge.

Preparation Time-20 minutes

Servings-2

Ingredients

For the dressing:

- 1 egg yolk
- ¼ ounce spicy mustard
- 2 ounces olive oil
- kosher salt
- 1/2 teaspoon chili powder
- 1 Pinch of cayenne pepper
- 1 teaspoon anchovy paste
- 1/4 ounce garlic, minced
- ½ ounce Lemon juice

For spicy shrimp:

- 6–8 ounces peeled and deveined medium shrimp
- 1/4 tsp chili powder
- 1 pinch of onion powder
- 1/2 teaspoon avocado oil
- 1 pinch of Kosher Salt
- 1 pinch ground pepper

For the salad:

- 48 ounces fresh spinach
- 1 small thinly sliced Cucumber
- 1 large thinly sliced carrot
- 1/2 sliced small peeled avocado
- 2 thinly sliced bell peppers
- 1 ½ ounces roasted almonds
- Gluten Free Croutons
- 4 ounces gluten-free bread
- 1 teaspoon olive oil
- 1/2 teaspoon garlic powder

Directions

1. Preheat oven to 450 degrees Fahrenheit

2. Whisk dressing **Ingredients** together in a mixing bowl and adjust seasoning according to taste. Wrap and store in refrigerator until ready to use.

3. Line a baking sheet with parchment paper. In a large bowl, toss shrimp in olive oil, chile powder, onion powder, avocado oil, salt and pepper. Lay the shrimp in one layer on the baking sheet.

4. Bake for 4-5 minutes per side until nicely browned and opaque. Remove shrimp from oven and let cool.

5. Line another baking sheet with parchment paper. In a bowl, toss bread crumbs in 1 teaspoon olive oil and garlic powder. Toss until coated and spread out on the baking sheet. Bake in oven for 5 minutes.

6. In a large serving bowl, combine spinach, vegetables, croutons and top it all with shrimp.

7. Toss **salad** in **salad** dressing and serve

24.Vegan Lo Mein

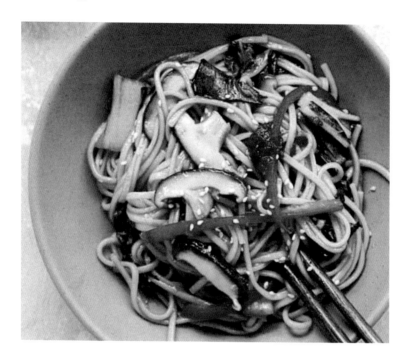

The vegans in your house will love the taste of this delicious and protein-packed treat. The sauce is sweet, savory and has a lovely spicy kick!

Preparation Time-20 minutes

Servings-2

Ingredients

- 7 ounces wholegrain pasta
- ½ ounce olive oil
- 1 minced clove garlic
- 8 ounces sliced mushrooms
- ½ red bell pepper
- 1 sliced carrot
- 1 ½ ounces white wine
- 2 ounces peas
- 2 ounces leafy greens like spinach

Sauce

- 2 ounces soy sauce
- 1/3 ounce maple syrup
- 2" knuckle of ginger, finely ground
- ¼ ounce Sriracha

Directions

Bring a pot of water to boil and cook pasta in water according to package **Directions**. Drain pasta.

Heat oil in a large pan on medium heat and sauté garlic, mushrooms, peppers and carrots in the oil. Stir often until vegetables are tender.

Pour wine into the pot and stir well. Stir in peas and leafy greens and let mixture simmer for 5 minutes

Whisk sauce **Ingredients** in a bowl until well combined.

Once vegetables are ready, transfer to a large bowl and mix in pasta, leafy greens and sauce. Toss all **Ingredients** until coated and serve.

25.Kale **salad** with Caesar dressing and avocado

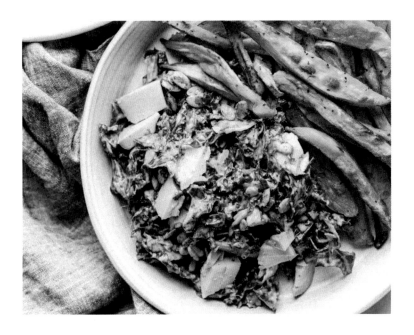

The key to a good kale **salad** is the preparation of the leaves beforehand. You want to soften and massage the kale leaves as much as possible for a pleasant consistency and taste.

Preparation Time-20 minutes

Servings-2

Ingredients

For the Dressing

- 1/2 ripened peeled and pitted avocado
- 2 ounces Creamy Caesar Dressing
- ½ lemon, juiced

For the salad

- 1 bunch curly green kale, washed, dried and tough stems removed
- 1 pinch sea salt
- 4 ounces carrots, shredded
- 2 ounces red onion, thinly sliced
- 8 ounces cherry tomatoes, cut in half
- 1 hard boiled egg, cut in half
- 1 ounce almonds, sliced

Directions

1. Combine avocado, lemon juice and **salad** dressing in a blender and process until smooth.

2. In a large mixing bowl, tear kale into small pieces and sprinkle with sea salt.

3. Massage the kale with your hands until they soften and wilt.

4. Take half of the kale and put in another bowl.

5. Evenly divide the rest of the **Ingredients** between the two bowls. Drizzle with **salad** dressing and serve.

26.Sheet pan salmon

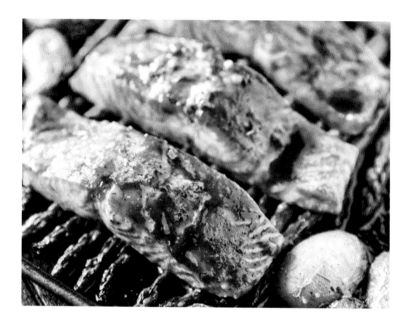

The refreshing splash of orange in this recipe gives the salmon an amazing flavor when you take your first bite. I have used lemon or lime juice in place of orange with great results.

Preparation Time-20 minutes

Servings-1

Ingredients

- 1 medium orange, skin and pit removed
- ½ ounce canola oil
- pepper
- salt
- 8 ounces thinly sliced kale leaves
- 4 ounces salmon fillet
- 6 ounces cooked farro

Directions

Heat oven to 450 degrees Fahrenheit. Line a baking sheet with parchment paper.

Separate orange into segments and squeeze out juice over a large mixing bowl. Stir in canola oil, salt and pepper.

Add kale leaves to the orange mixture and toss until fully coated. Transfer mixture from bowl to the prepared baking sheet and spread out evenly.

Sprinkle salmon fillet with salt and pepper and place on top of the mixture in the baking sheet.

Roast salmon for 7-10 minutes until it flakes easily with a fork.

Place farro in the microwave and cook on high for 30-second intervals until heated through.

Arrange hot farro evenly on a serving dish and place salmon and vegetables on the farro. Serve and enjoy!

27.Jalapeno popper chicken

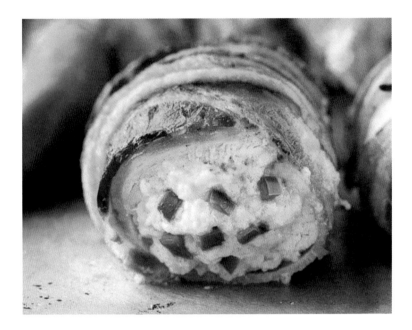

These poppers are a tasty treat for social gatherings and potlucks. I like to make a jalapeno and cream cheese dip for extra zip!

Preparation Time-10 minutes

Servings-4

Ingredients

- 4 x 4-ounce chicken breasts, flattened to ½" thick
- 2 jalapeño peppers

- 4 ounces softened cream cheese
- 4 ounces shredded cheddar cheese
- 8 strips bacon

Directions

Preheat oven to 375 degrees Fahrenheit

Evenly split the jalapeño peppers, cream cheese and cheddar cheese on the chicken breasts.

Wrap chicken around the filling and wrap the chicken in two pieces of bacon each.

Secure with a toothpick and place in an oven-safe baking dish.

Bake for 30-35 minutes until chicken is no longer pink inside and bacon is crispy.

28.Sheet pan dinner

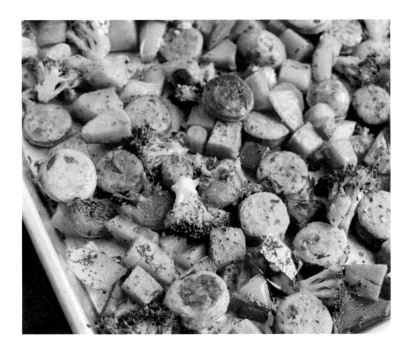

You can enjoy this recipe as a meal on its own or as a side for salmon, beef or chicken. Add a little cornstarch in water to the dressing to thicken it up.

Preparation Time-10 minutes

Servings-4

Ingredients

- 6 pork sausages
- 6 slices of bacon, chopped
- 1 diced onion
- 1 head of cauliflower, diced
- 32 ounces Brussels sprouts, diced
- 1 teaspoon salt
- 1 teaspoon turmeric
- 1 teaspoon black pepper
- 1 teaspoon ghee
- ½ ounce coconut oil
- 3 ounces mayonnaise

Directions

1. Pre-heat oven to 400 degrees Fahrenheit.

2. Toss onion, cauliflower, Brussels sprouts, salt, turmeric, ghee and black pepper in a large mixing bowl. Line two baking sheets with parchment paper. Divide the onion mixture between the two baking sheets

3. Slice into sausages ¾" way down and repeat until it resembles an accordion. Place sausages in the vegetables on the baking sheets.

4. Spread bacon pieces evenly among the vegetables on the baking sheets.

5. Roast for 30 minutes. Drizzle dressing over the sausages and broil for 5 minutes.

29.Black Bean and Corn **salad**

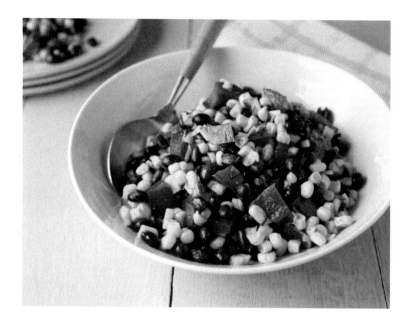

This **salad** makes a lovely side dish for any protein-packed meal. You can also enjoy this **salad** on its own as an afternoon snack.

Preparation Time-10 minutes

Servings-2

Ingredients

- 1 x 15 ½ ounce can drained black beans, rinsed
- 7 ½ ounces canned sweet corn, drained and rinsed

- 1 red onion, thinly sliced
- 2 spring onions, thinly sliced
- 2 ½ ounces couscous
- 4 ounces vegetable broth
- 1 ounce olive oil
- 1 juiced lemon
- 1/3 ounce cumin
- 1/3 ounce paprika powder
- 1/3 ounce chili flakes
- 1 chopped clove garlic

Directions

Pour boiling water into broth and pour over couscous in a large mixing bowl until it just covers it. Soak for 5-10 minutes.

Add the rest of the **Ingredients** to the couscous and mix well. Serve and enjoy!

30.Ground beef veggie skillet

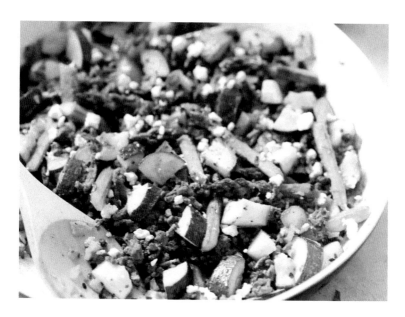

This recipe is delicious on its own and very filling. You can also use this dish as a filling for a whole wheat tortilla.

Preparation Time-10 minutes

Servings-4

Ingredients

- 1 ounce extra virgin olive oil
- 16 ounces extra-lean ground beef
- 1 minced clove garlic

- 4 ounces diced onions
- 4 ounces diced red bell peppers
- 8 ounces asparagus, cut into thirds
- 1 medium quartered zucchini
- 1 teaspoon Dijon mustard
- ½ teaspoon dried oregano
- 2 ounces tomato passata
- ⅛ teaspoon red pepper, crushed
- salt
- freshly ground black pepper
- ½ ounce crumbled feta cheese
- fresh parsley, chopped

Directions

1. Heat oil in a large frying pan on medium high heat

2. Add beef and garlic to the oil and cook for 7-8 minutes until beef is evenly browned. Break up the meat chunks with a wooden spoon as you cook.

3. Remove mixture from frying pan and add onions to the drippings. Cook for 3-4 minutes until tender.

4. Add a little more olive oil to the pan if needed and sauté zucchini and asparagus for 3-5 minutes until tender.

5. Replace ground beef and onion to the frying pan and mix all **Ingredients** well.

6. Add mustard, passata, oregano, red pepper, salt and pepper and mix well.

7. Serve topped with parsley and feta cheese.

Conclusion

From black bean **salad** to vegetable skillets, this recipe book has something that everyone will enjoy. Whether you are meat eater, a vegetarian or following a protein-rich diet, you will be able to find a simple and satisfying dish within these pages. Try an ideal protein recipe today and reap the benefits of a healthy lifestyle!